Freestyle 2018

Quick, Easy and Delicious Points Recipes for You to Shed Excess Weight, Regain Confidence and Have a Happy Life

By Dona Tommy

Contents

Chapter 1: Essentials of WW Freestyle Program

According to a recent survey performed by US News, the Weight Watchers Freestyle program is voted as one of the most highly effective dietary programs out there, designed to trim down excess body weight while keeping you healthy!

This alone is an awe-inspiring feat, mainly because this program got this adulation while fighting with hundreds of other "Top" diets out there!

But word of mouth won't be enough to convince you to follow the diet right? So, let me give you a brief breakdown.

Let's start with...

A Brief History of WW Freestyle Program

The Weight Watchers Program is perhaps one of the unique dietary programs to ever come to fruition because this particular program is not the labor of thousands of "Money-Hungry" scientists trying to figure out the next "breakthrough"!

Instead, this was the brainchild of a very humble and simple-minded homemaker named Jean Nidetech who was looking for a solution to overcome "Obesity."

Jean herself was an individual who consistently suffered from the hardships of obesity, and the Weight Watchers diet is the birth child of her constant struggle to control her food lust and trim down her fat.

During her exploratory journey of self-discovery, she took multiple steps and tried her best to trim down her fat by experimenting with a lot of different diets!

Perhaps it's safe to say that the Weight Watchers Program is the love labor seeded by her struggles that led her to have a very important epiphany that would, later on, form the foundation of the program.

Upon reaching the end of her initial weight loss journey, she soon realized that just "loosing" weight isn't the solution to obesity, as people might quickly start eating more and gain double the weight that they have lost!

She soon realized that in the long run, dieting isn't the solution to the obesity problem. In fact, according to her acute judgment, the primary source of the problem was "Lack of control."

Keeping that in mind, she eventually took the help of her friends and families and started the "Weight Watchers' Organization" to help other obese and likeminded people who were looking for help.

The "Points" system implemented in the Weight Watchers program was very carefully designed to enforce a sense of dietary control that was easily accessible to anyone, which eventually brought the program into the limelight.

The updated version of the Weight Watchers Program that we follow today is the "Weight Watchers Freestyle" program that uses an updated "SmartPoints" system!

But as you can see now, the revolutionary idea had its seed planted back in the 1920s!

The Basics of Weight Watchers Program

Before going into the concepts of the new "Weight Watchers Freestyle," it is of paramount that you have a good understanding of the original diet, which makes up the foundation of the new one.

So, we will use the original Weight Watchers program as our starting point.

Unlike most so-called "professional" diets out there, the Weight Watchers doesn't ask you to follow a rigorous and concise dietary regime that would have you to eliminate every single food that you love!

Instead, it implements a very meticulously crafted "Points" system that encourages you to make healthy life and dietary choices with the help of "Assigning" a set number of points to each different food groups and ingredients.

At first, this might sound a bit strange but bear with me, and everything will clear up eventually.

Throughout the years since the conception of the very first Weight Watchers program, there have been numerous updates to this points system and the one that we are following is called the "SmartPoints" system, which is an overhauled version of the previous "PointsPlus" one.

In 2018 though, the Weight Watchers organization took another bold step and update their already popular "SmartPoints" system further through the introduction of the "Freestyle Program."

The Freestyle Program is an extension to the regular Weight Watchers program that brings about some fresh changes.

Keep in mind that the Freestyle program still follows the previously created SmartPoint system. However, the number of points assigned to specific food groups are significantly slashed down the 0 in the "Freestyle" program.

In the previous program, each was assigned a set number of daily points depending on various factors such as sex, height, and others (including your target weight to be lost)

The Freestyle program followed the same method but tweaked the formula slightly to ensure that the owners can enjoy maximum benefit from this diet.

How the Freestyle Program Works?

As you may have already guessed, the beating heart of the Weight Watchers program is the "SmartPoints" system itself.

So, let me break down the points system to you to give you a better understanding of the Science behind the program.

Keep in mind that the Freestyle program uses a revamped version of the "SmartPoint" program. Therefore I will explain the SmartPoints system here.

A simple formula for calculating the Smartpoints of your meal is done using the formula below.

Points = (Calories + (Fat x 4) – (Fiber x 10))/50

However, if you want greater accuracy, then you can always refer to the provided list of the common ingredients (and their SP) in the section below.

As for calculating your daily SmartPoints limit, there are some fantastic calculators out there that will help you to achieve that. Two good examples are
http://www.healthyweightforum.org/eng/calculators/ww:points:allowed/
or http://www.calculator.net/weight:watchers:points:calculator.html

To give you an idea though, let us follow an example where we assume that you 20 years old male and have a weight of 70kgs with a height of 5 feet and your target is to lose 10 kg, and then your allocated SP will be 30.

However, the best way to calculate your Daily and Weekly Allowance is still through the official Weight Watchers App provided upon availing your membership.

But if you want to experiment with the program for free, then the websites mentioned above will be able to help you while the following apps will help you as well.

- Ultimate Food Diary App (This app is the only one that has been updated to provide services that resemble the Freestyle meal plan)
- iTrackBites (This is yet another app that is very close to the official WW app. However, this did not support the Freestyle program at the time of writing, but was supposed to be updated very soon)

This means that you are allowed to eat as much as you want as long as you are not crossing your daily point limit.

Differences between New and Old Freestyle Program

As mentioned before, the following are the most crucial changes that differ the new "Freestyle" program from the old one.

- **Exclusive "0" Point Foods:** This is perhaps the most significant change in the new program. Various ingredients and food items that had a significant number of SmartPoints accompanying them have been completely cut down to Zero. This gives you greater freedom when choosing your meal and designing your plans.

- **The SmartPoints:** The updated Freestyle program will still use the same method of calculation. However, your daily SmartPoint allocation will change a bit to balance out the new foods that are all zeroed out now. If you are already a member of the Weight Watchers program, then you may be able to do this with through their designated app, or you may use the apps mentioned in the previous section.

- **Weekly Point Allowance:** Despite having a change in your daily point allowance, the weekly allowance will remain the same. This means that you will be able to include more food and adjust your plans with greater flexibility.

- **Rollover Points:** This is yet another feature that comes as an exclusive to the Weight Watchers Freestyle program! The "Roll Over" system allows you to transfer a maximum of 4 unused daily points from the current week to the next week if you need! So for example, if you have a current Weekly limit of 120 Smart Points and you used only 116 SmartPoint in the previous week, then you have 4 Roll Over points! Which means in the coming week, you have 124 SmartPoints to consider The Roll Over Points is a great strategy that helps to prepare you for an upcoming event.

PROS AND CONS OF FREESTYLE PROGRAM

Like every diet out there, there are some pros and cons that you should consider before embarking on your journey!

- Unlike most diets, Weight Watchers won't ask you to follow a very strict diet routine that would eliminate all of your favorite food
- Through the meetings and membership, offers you will enjoy and receive various cooking advices and nutritional tips
- The Weight Watchers is not limited to adults only! Even kids and teenagers can follow a lighter version of the diet to stay fit!
- The Smart Points system encourages to maintain your portions which will allow you to gradually and steadily lose your weight
- Through FitPoints, exercise is largely encouraged which helps to maintain a nice physique

However

- Group meetings are an integral part of the Weight Watchers process and some individuals might feel a bit uncomfortable sharing their personal information in front of other people
- Keeping track of the SmartPoints might become slightly tedious if you don't have enough patience
- Weekly weight loss progress might discourage you a little bit because Weight Loss with Weight Watchers takes time to make a significant impact

The Old SmartPoints Food List

Below is a list of the most common ingredients alongside their associated Smart Point for your convenience.

Food with 0 SP

- Coffee
- Banana
- Apple
- Strawberries
- Chicken Breast
- Salad
- Blueberries
- Grapes

- Tomatoes
- Watermelon
- Egg White
- Lettuce
- Deli Sliced Turkey Breast
- Baby Carrots
- Orange
- Cucumber
- Broccoli
- Water
- Green Beans
- Pineapple
- Corn On The Cob (medium)
- Cherries
- Cantaloupe
- Spinach
- Fresh Fruit
- Raspberries
- Shrimp
- Asparagus
- Celery
- Cherry Tomatoes
- Carrots
- Yogurt
- Peach
- Sweet Red Potatoes
- Pear
- Salsa
- Tuna
- Diet Coke
- Mushrooms
- Onions
- Black Beans
- Blackberries
- Zucchini
- Grape Tomatoes
- Mixed Berries
- Grapefruit
- Nectarine
- Mango
- Mustard

Food with 1 SP

- Sugar
- Almond Milk
- Egg
- Guacamole
- Half and Half
- Salad Dressing

Food with 2 SP

- Cream
- Avocado
- 1 Slice Of Bread
- Scrambled Egg with milk/ butter
- Luncheon Meat, deli sliced or ham (2 ounces)
- 2 t tablespoon of Hummus

Food with 3 SP

- Milk Skimmed
- One tablespoon of Mayonnaise

- Chocolate Chip Cookies
- Sweet potatoes ½ a cup
- 3 ounce of boneless Pork Chop
- 1 ounce of flour Tortilla
- Italian Salad Dressing 2 tablespoon
- Three slices of cooked Turkey Bacon
- 1 cup of Cottage Cheese
- An ounce of crumbled Feta

Food with 4 SP

- Olive Oil
- American Cheese 1 slice
- Low Fat Milk 1%, 1 Cup
- Cheddar Cheese 1 ounce
- Red Wine 5 ounce
- ¼ cup of Almond
- 5 ounce of White Wine
- Tortilla Chips 1 ounce
- Shredded Cheddar Cheese
- One tablespoon of honey
- 102 ounce of English Muffin
- Mashed Potatoes

Food with 5 SP

- Butter
- 3 Slices of Cooked Bacon
- Reduced Fat Milk 1 Cup
- Cooked Oatmeal 1 cup
- Plain Baked Potato, 6 ounce
- Regular Beer, 12 ounce
- 1 cup of cooked regular/ whole wheat pasta

- Hamburger Bun
- Ranch Salad Dressing
- Any type of Bagel (2 ounce)
- 1 cup of Spaghetti

Food With 6+ SP

- White Rice (6)
- Brown Rice (6)
- Peanut Butter 2 tablespoon (6)
- 1 Whole Cup Of Milk (7)
- 20 ounce of French Fries (13)
- 1 cup of cooked Quinoa (6)

NEW "0" SMARTPOINT INGREDIENTS

- Peas such as chickpeas, sugar snap peas, black-eyed, etc.
- Beans such as black beans, kidney beans, pinto beans, fat-free refried beans, soybeans, sprouts, etc.
- Lentils
- Corn such as baby corn, sweet corn, corn on the cob
- Skinless Chicken Breast
- Skinless Turkey Breast
- Tofu
- Egg and Egg Whites
- Fish and Shellfish
- Yogurt
- Lean Ground Beef
- Non-Fat and Plain Greek Yogurt
- All Fruits
- All Vegetables

To give you a more detailed look at the list, the following now hold a 0 SmartPoint value.

- Yogurt
- Plain Yogurt
- Greek Yogurt
- Watermelon
- Watercress
- Water Chestnuts
- Stir Fried Vegetables
- Mixed Vegetables
- Sticks of Vegetables
- Turnips
- Turkey Breast
- Turkey Breast Tenderloin
- Ground Turkey Breast
- Tomato
- Tomato Sauce
- Tofu
- Taro
- Tangerine
- Tangelo
- Starfruit
- Winter and Summer Squash
- Spinach
- Shellfish
- Shallots
- Scallions
- Sauerkraut
- Chicken Satay
- Sashimi
- Salsa
- Salad
- Lentils
- Lime
- Lettuce
- Litchi
- Mangoes
- Mung Dal
- Mushroom Caps
- Nectarine
- Okra
- Onions
- Orange
- Parsley
- Pea Shoot
- Peaches
- Pear
- Pepper
- Pickles
- Pineapple
- Plums
- Pomegranate Seeds
- Pomelo
- Pumpkin
- Pumpkin Puree
- Radish
- Salad Mixed Greens
- Salad Three Bean
- Lemon Zest
- Leek
- Kiwifruit
- Jicama
- Jerk Chicken Breast
- Jackfruit
- Heart of Palm
- Guava
- Mixed Baby Greens
- Ginger Root
- Grape Fruit
- Fruit Cup
- Fruit Cocktail
- Fish Fillet
- Fruit
- Fish

- Figs
- Fennel
- Escarole
- Endive
- Egg Whites
- Eggs
- Apples
- Arrowroot
- Applesauce
- Artichoke
- Artichoke Hearts
- Bamboo Shoots
- Banana
- Beans
- Beets
- Blueberries
- Blackberries
- Broccoli
- Brussels
- Cabbage
- Carrots
- Cauliflower
- Cherries
- Chicken Breast
- Clementine
- Cucumber
- Dragon Fruit
- Egg Substitute
- Dates

And a few more.

The Relationship between Weight Loss And SmartPoints

Perhaps this is the main reason as to why you are even reading this book right?
Well, the idea behind losing weight through the Weight Watchers Freestyle Diet isn't as straightforward as it may seem!
Mainly because the core aim of this diet is to not only act as a means of "Losing Excess Fat" but also as a means to "Keep You Under Control" in the long run.
This program is not designed to be a temporary solution, but rather a long-term process that helps you to stay fit and lean for the rest of your journey.
In one of the previous section, I have already explained the basic concepts of "HOW" you can calculate your weekly allocated SmartPoints limit.
Since this weekly limit largely depends on multiple parameters such as your current weight, target weight, time, age, sex, etc. the weekly SmartPoint limit largely varies from person to person, so there's no "One" answer as to how much weight you can lose within a week.

It will ultimately depend on how much effort you are willing to put into the diet and how strictly you will follow it.

However, if you move at a good pace and adhere to your allocated SmartPoints limit, then you will quickly trim down 1-2 pounds of unwanted fat each week!

And the best part?

As long as you are sticking to the program, those unwanted and lost fats won't even come back thanks to the carefully thought out system!

Amazing Tips for a Successful Freestyle Program

- Make sure to learn how to maintain and control your portions. Having a good understanding of standard measurements such as ounce, cups, etc. are crucial when creating a meal plan. You don't want to overshoot your meal portions as it might lead to an unsatisfactory result.
- Although the SmartPoints for the recipes is roughly calculated in this book using the provided outline (in the appendix), it is still recommended that you learn how to figure the SmartPoints by yourself.
- Make sure to skip "Diet" soft drinks. While they might be free from unwanted calories, they still pack a good load of artificial sweeteners, which may lead to various medical issues.
- While practicing your portion control, you should never skip on exercise! Even if it is for 5-10 minutes, you should try not to avoid a short daily exercise routine.
- When you are eating, always try to split the meals if you have someone else to share your meals with. This will allow you to lower down both your calorie and point intake.
- Using the SP list found in the end, experiment with various ingredients and recipes using this book as a source of inspiration and create your very own meals!

A NOTE ON HOW MUCH IT COSTS

Since this diet does not provide a specific dietary regime for you to follow, the actual "Cost" of the food ultimately depends on you!

The flexibility of the diet allows you to carve up your meal plan depending on your budget.

However, if you are looking for an online membership or are interested in joining the meetings, then you are to pay a minimal signup fee.

At the time of writing, the online membership had a fee of 17.5$ per month, which had an additional 29.95$ initiation fee.

On the other hand, you can also go for In-Person meetings with unlimited access for $39.95 which has its perks as well.

So, for the official support from the Weight Watchers community, you may expect a bill of 50-60$.

Keep in mind that these numbers are subject to change, and it is highly recommended that visit www.weightwatchers.com to get an updated value of their current plans.

But everything said and done, the plan ultimately depends on you!

The only thing to keep in mind is to "not" cross your daily SmartPoint limit.

In terms following the Freestyle Diet, the most important thing to remember is not to exceed your weekly allocated SmartPoints limit.

CHAPTER 2: BREAKFAST RECIPES

1. MOUTHWATERING EGG AND RICOTTA BREAD

(Prepping time: 5 minutes\ Cooking time: 10 minutes |For 4 servings\SmartPoints:3)

Ingredients

- 4 medium whole eggs
- 4 tablespoon of skimmed milk
- 4 slices of whole meal bread
- Cooking spray as needed
- 9 ounce cherry tomatoes
- 9 ounce Ricotta cheese

Directions

1. Crack the eggs in an bowl and beat them with a seasoning of black pepper
2. Take a shallow dish and add breads in layer
3. Pour the egg mix over the bread and coat well
4. Take a large non-stick frying pan and place it over medium heat
5. Mist with cooking spray
6. Fry the breads in batches giving 2-3 minutes per sides until the breads are golden brown
7. Cut the fried slices in half and keep them on the side
8. Add tomatoes to the same pan and stir for 2-3 minutes
9. Serve bread with tomatoes and ricotta. Enjoy!

Nutrition Values (Per Serving)

- Calories: 254
- Fat: 9g
- Carbohydrates: 34g
- Protein: 8g

2. Berry And Almond Smoothie

(Prepping time: 10 minutes\ Cooking time: 0 minutes |For 4 servings\SmartPoints:2)

Ingredients

- 1 cup of blueberries, frozen
- 1 whole banana
- ½ a cup of almond milk
- 1 tablespoon of almond butter
- Water as needed

Directions

1. Add the listed ingredients to your blender
2. Blend them well until you have a smooth texture
3. Chill and serve!

Nutrition Values (Per Serving)

- Calories: 321
- Fat: 11g
- Carbohydrates: 55g
- Protein: 5g

3. Exotic Pineapple Juice

(Prepping time: 10 minutes\ Cooking time: 0 minutes |For 3 servings\SmartPoints:4)

Ingredients

- 4 cups of fresh pineapple, chopped
- 1 pinch of salt
- 1 and a ½ cup of water

Directions

1. Add the listed ingredients to a HIGH-SPEED blender
2. Pulse until you have a smooth mixture
3. Strain the juice through a strainer and serve in 3 glasses
4. Enjoy!

Nutrition Values (Per Serving)

- Calories: 82
- Fat: 0.2g
- Carbohydrates: 21g
- Protein: 21g

4. ORIGINAL ARABIC FATTOUSH SALAD

(Prepping time: 15 minutes\ Cooking time: 2-3 minutes |For 4 servings\SmartPoints:2)

Ingredients

- 1 whole wheat pita bread
- 1 large English cucumber, diced
- 2 cup grape tomatoes, halved
- ½ of a medium red onion, finely diced
- ¾ cup of fresh parsley, chopped
- ¾ cup of mint leaves, chopped
- 1 clove of garlic, minced
- ¼ cup of fat free feta cheese, crumbled
- 1 tablespoon of olive oil
- 1 teaspoon of ground sumac
- Juice from ½ a lemon
- Salt and pepper as needed

Directions

1. Lightly mist the pita bread with cooking spray
2. Season with salt
3. Toast until crisp and has a golden brown texture
4. Take a large bowl and add the rest of the ingredients, (except feta)
5. Top with diced pita and feta cheese
6. Serve and enjoy!

Nutrition Values (Per Serving)

- Calories: 86
- Fat: 3g
- Carbohydrates: 9g
- Protein: 9g

5. Healthy Cauliflower Salad

(Prepping time: 8 minutes\ Cooking time: 0 minutes |For 3 servings\SmartPoints:1)

Ingredients

- 1 head of cauliflower, broken into florets
- 1 small onion, chopped
- 1/8 cup of extra virgin olive oil
- ¼ cup of apple cider vinegar
- ½ a teaspoon of sea salt
- ½ a teaspoon of black pepper
- ¼ cup of dried cranberries
- ¼ cup of pumpkin seeds

Directions

1. Wash the cauliflower and break it up into small florets
2. Transfer to a bowl
3. Whisk oil, vinegar, salt and pepper in another bowl
4. Add pumpkin seeds, cranberries to the bowl with dressing
5. Mix well and pour the dressing over the cauliflower
6. Add onions and toss
7. Chill and serve
8. Enjoy!

Nutrition Values (Per Serving)

- Calories: 163
- Fat: 11g
- Carbohydrates: 16g
- Protein: 3g

6. Early Morning 3 Ingredient Pancake

(Prepping time: 15 minutes\ Cooking time: 10 minutes |For 4 servings\SmartPoints:2)

Ingredients

- 1 small ripe banana
- 1 medium sized egg
- 2 tablespoon of whole meal self-rising flour
- Cooking spray as needed

Directions

1. Take a medium sized bowl and add bananas, mash using fork
2. Whisk in eggs, flour and mix well until properly combined
3. Allow the mix to sit for about 5 minutes
4. Take a non-stick frying pan and grease with oil
5. Heat up pan over medium-heat and spoon 2 tablespoon of the prepared batter
6. Cook each side for 2 minutes until both sides of the cake are golden
7. Repeat with the remaining batter until all batter has been used up
8. Serve and enjoy!

Nutrition Values (Per Serving)

- Calories: 139
- Fat: 6g
- Carbohydrates: 18g
- Protein: 3g

7. Ham and Egg Muffins

(Prepping time: 10 minutes\ Cooking time: 20 minutes |For 12 servings\SmartPoints:3)

Ingredients

- 12 whole eggs
- 12 slices of ham
- Paprika
- Pepper and salt as needed

Directions

1. Pre-heat your oven to 375 degree Fahrenheit
2. Take 12 muffin tins and line with 1 ham
3. Crack an egg into each muffin tin
4. Season muffin with paprika, salt and paprika
5. Place in your oven and bake for 20 minutes
6. Enjoy once ready!

Nutrition Values (Per Serving)

- Calories: 210
- Fat: 6g
- Carbohydrates: 27g
- Protein: 14g

8. Italian Baked Egg

(Prepping time: 10 minutes\ Cooking time: 20 minutes |For 4 servings\SmartPoints:7)

Ingredients

- 2 cup marinara sauce
- ¼ cup fresh basil, chopped
- 4 large eggs
- ½ a cup of parmesan cheese, grated
- ¼ teaspoon of red pepper flakes

Directions

1. Pre-heat your oven to 350 degree Fahrenheit
2. Place oven rack in the middle position
3. Pour marinara sauce into a square baking dish and sprinkle basil
4. Make 4 narrow wells and crack an egg into the center of each well
5. Sprinkle eggs with parmesan cheese and red pepper flakes
6. Bake for 18-20 minutes
7. Divide the sauce and eggs amongst 4 bowls
8. Server and enjoy!

Nutrition Values (Per Serving)

- Calories: 112
- Fat: 4g
- Carbohydrates: 9g
- Protein: 11g

9. Quinoa And Date Flurry

(Prepping time: 10 minutes\ Cooking time: 15 minutes |For 2 servings\SmartPoints:6)

Ingredients

- 1 date, pitted and chopped finely
- ½ a cup of red quinoa, dried
- 1 cup of unsweetened almond milk
- 1/8 teaspoon of vanilla extract
- ¼ cup of fresh strawberries, hulled and sliced
- 1/8 teaspoon of ground cinnamon

Directions

1. Take a pan and place it over low heat
2. Add quinoa, almond milk, cinnamon, vanilla and cook for about 15 minutes, making sure to keep stirring it from time to time
3. Garnish with strawberries and enjoy!

Nutrition Values (Per Serving)

- Calories: 195
- Fat: 4.4g
- Carbohydrates: 32g
- Protein: 7g

10. Quinoa And Black Bean Salad

(Prepping time: 5 minutes\ Cooking time: 15 minutes |For 6 servings\SmartPoints:5)

Ingredients

- 1 cup of uncooked quinoa
- 1 can of 15 ounce black beans, drained and rinsed
- 1/3 cup of cilantro, chopped
- 1 tablespoon of olive oil
- 1 clove garlic, minced
- Juice from 1 lime
- Salt and pepper as needed

Directions

7. Cook quinoa according to package instructions
8. Transfer quinoa to a medium bowl and allow it to cool for 10 minutes
9. Add rest of the ingredients and toss
10. Serve and enjoy!

Nutrition Values (Per Serving)

- Calories: 188
- Fat: 4g
- Carbohydrates: 29g
- Protein: 8g

11. Simple Bowl Of Berry And Yogurt

(Prepping time: 10 minutes\ Cooking time: 0 minutes |For 6 servings\SmartPoints:3)

Ingredients

- 3 cups of fat-free plain yogurt
- 1 cup of fresh raspberries
- 1 cup of fresh blueberries
- 2 teaspoon of raw honey

Directions

1. Take a bowl and mix honey and yogurt
2. Top with raspberries and blueberries and stir
3. Serve immediately and enjoy!

Nutrition Values (Per Serving)

- Calories: 100
- Fat: 0.4g
- Carbohydrates: 17g
- Protein: 8g

12. EXCELLENT GRANOLA BOWL

(Prepping time: 5 minutes\ Cooking time: 25 minutes |For 6 servings\SmartPoints:2)

Ingredients

- 1 ounce Porridge oats
- 2 teaspoon of maple syrup
- Cooking spray as needed
- 4 medium bananas
- 4 pots of Caramel Layered Fromage Frais
- 5 ounce Fresh Fruit Salad such as strawberries, blueberries and raspberries
- ¼ ounce pumpkin seeds
- ¼ ounce sunflower seeds
- ¼ ounce dry Chia seeds
- ¼ ounce Desiccated coconut

Directions

1. Preheat your oven to 302 degree Fahrenheit
2. Line up baking tray with baking paper
3. Take a large bowl and add oats, seeds, maple syrup
4. Spread the mixture out on the baking tray
5. Mix with coconut oil spray and bake for 20 minutes, making sure to keep stirring it from time to time
6. Sprinkle coconut at the 15 minutes point
7. Remove from the oven and spread out on cold baking tray
8. Slice bananas and layer in a bowl with Fromage Frais
9. Sprinkle granola on top and serve with the berries. Enjoy!

Nutrition Values (Per Serving)

- Calories: 446
- Fat: 29g
- Carbohydrates: 37g
- Protein: 13g

13. Healthy Banana Smoothie

(Prepping time: 5 minutes\ Cooking time: 0 minutes |For 2 servings\SmartPoints:2)

Ingredients

- 1 whole large banana
- 2 cups of kale, chopped
- ½ a cup of light unsweetened almond milk
- 1 tablespoon of flax seeds

Directions

1. Add the listed ingredients to your blender
2. Blend them well until you have a smooth texture
3. Chill and serve!

Nutrition Values (Per Serving)

- Calories: 311
- Fat: 7g
- Carbohydrates: 56g
- Protein: 12g

14. Delicious Apple Porridge

(Prepping time: 10 minutes\ Cooking time: 5 minutes |For 2 servings\SmartPoints:5)

Ingredients

- 1 large apple, peeled, cored and grated
- 1 cup unsweetened almond milk
- 1 and a ½ tablespoon of sunflower seeds
- 1/8 cup of fresh blueberries
- ¼ teaspoon of vanilla extract

Directions

1. Add sunflower seeds, almond milk, vanilla extract and apples in a large sized pan
2. Place the pan over medium-low heat
3. Cook for 5 minutes making sure to keep stirring it well
4. Transfer to serving bowls and enjoy!

Nutrition Values (Per Serving)

- Calories: 123
- Fat: 1.3g
- Carbohydrates:23g
- Protein: 4g

15. Spinach And Scrambled Egg

(Prepping time: 10 minutes\ Cooking time: 10 minutes |For 6 servings\SmartPoints:1)

Ingredients

- 1 and a ½ tablespoon of extra virgin olive oil
- ½ a cup of 2% sharp cheddar cheese
- 1 teaspoon of salt
- 1 teaspoon of pepper
- 1 clove garlic, crushed and minced
- ½ a red onion, diced
- 3 cups of organic baby spinach
- 1 organic tomato, diced
- 6 large whole eggs

Directions

1. Take a large bowl and whisk in salt, pepper and eggs
2. Mix well
3. Take a large non-stick skillet and place it over medium high head
4. Add oil and allow the oil to heat up
5. Add garlic, onions and Saute for 5 minutes
6. Stir in tomatoes and Saute for 3 minutes
7. Stir in spinach and cook for 2 minutes more
8. Pour eggs and cook for 5 minutes
9. Serve and enjoy!

Nutrition Values (Per Serving)

- Calories: 219
- Fat: 15g
- Carbohydrates: 3g
- Protein: 16g

16. Supreme Egg Benedict

(Prepping time: 20 minutes\ Cooking time: 10 minutes |For 4 servings\SmartPoints:7)

Ingredients

- 1 tablespoon of white wine
- 4 large eggs
- 4 slices of Canadian bacon
- ¼ cup of fat free plain Greek yogurt
- ¼ cup low calorie mayonnaise
- 1 teaspoon of Dijon mustard
- ½ a teaspoon of lemon zest
- 1 teaspoon of lemon juice, freshly squeezed
- 2 teaspoon of unsalted butter
- 2 light whole grain English muffins, split and toasted
- 1 medium tomato, cut into 4 thick slices

Directions

1. Take a large skillet and fill it halfway with water
2. Bring to a boil over medium-high heat
3. Stir in vinegar and lower down the heat to low, bring to a simmer
4. Break eggs into the boiling water one at a time and cook for 4 minutes until the egg whites are set
5. Remove the eggs using a slotted spoon and let them drain, discard the water
6. Wipe the skillet and place it over medium-high heat
7. Add Canadian bacon and cook for 1 minute each side
8. Take a small microwave safe bowl and whisk in yogurt, mayonnaise, mustard, lemon juice, lemon zest .Microwave for 30 seconds
9. Stir in butter until melted
10. Place a slice of tomato, Canadian bacon, egg on top of your English muffin half. Drizzle 2 tablespoon of sauce. Serve and enjoy!

Nutrition Values (Per Serving)

- Calories: 478
- Fat: 38g
- Carbohydrates: 15g
- Protein: 22g

17. Mesmerizing Orange and Onion Salad

(Prepping time: 10 minutes\ Cooking time: 0 minutes |For 3 servings\SmartPoints:2)

Ingredients

- 6 large orange
- 3 tablespoon of red wine vinegar
- 6 tablespoon of olive oil
- 1 teaspoon of dried oregano
- 1 red onion, thinly sliced
- 1 cup olive oil
- ¼ cup of fresh chives, chopped
- Ground black pepper

Directions

1. Peel the orange and cut each of them in 4-5 crosswise slices
2. Transfer the oranges to a shallow dish
3. Drizzle vinegar, olive oil and sprinkle oregano
4. Toss
5. Chill for 30 minutes
6. Arrange sliced onion and black olives on top
7. Decorate with additional sprinkle of chives and fresh grind of pepper
8. Serve and enjoy!

Nutrition Values (Per Serving)

- Calories: 120
- Fat: 6g
- Carbohydrates: 20g
- Protein: 2g

18. Smiling Coffee Banana Smoothie

(Prepping time: 10 minutes\ Cooking time: 0 minutes |For 2 servings\SmartPoints:5)

Ingredients

- 1 cup of chilled brewed coffee
- 1 and a ½ banana, cut into chunks
- 1 cup of non-fat plain Greek yogurt
- 1 tablespoon of ground flax seed
- 2 teaspoon of agave nectar
- ½ a teaspoon of ground cinnamon
- ¼ teaspoon of grated nutmeg
- 6 ice cubes

Directions

1. Add all the listed ingredients to a blender and blend well until the mixture is smooth
2. Serve chilled and enjoy!

Nutrition Values (Per Serving)

- Calories: 126
- Fat: 1g
- Carbohydrates: 21g
- Protein: 10g

19. A Mean Green Vegetable Smoothie

(Prepping time: 10 minutes\ Cooking time: 0 minutes |For 4 servings\SmartPoints:1)

Ingredients

- 1 cup green cabbage, chopped
- ½ a cup of fresh spinach
- 3 cups of chilled water
- 1 cup of broccoli florets, chopped
- 1 cup of small green bell pepper, seeded and chopped
- 2 and a ½ drops of liquid stevia

Directions

1. Add the listed ingredients to a blender
2. Pulse until you have smooth mixture
3. Transfer to serving glass and serve chilled
4. Enjoy!

Nutrition Values (Per Serving)

- Calories: 25
- Fat: 0.2g
- Carbohydrates: 5.3g
- Protein: 2g

20. Avocado And Cilantro Delight

(Prepping time: 10 minutes\ Cooking time: 0 minutes |For 6 servings\SmartPoints:2)

Ingredients

- 2 avocados, peeled , pitted and diced
- 1 sweet onion, chopped
- 1 green bell pepper, chopped
- 1 large ripe tomato, chopped
- ¼ cup of fresh cilantro, chopped
- ½ a lime, juiced
- Salt and pepper as needed

Directions

1. Take a medium sized bowl and add onion, tomato, avocados, bell pepper, lime and cilantro
2. Give the whole mixture a toss
3. Season accordingly and serve chilled
4. Enjoy!

Nutrition Values (Per Serving)

- Calories: 126
- Fat: 10g
- Carbohydrates: 10g
- Protein: 2g

21. Whole Wheat Apple And Cinnamon Pancakes

(Prepping time: 10 minutes\ Cooking time: 10 minutes |For 2 servings\SmartPoints:5)

Ingredients

- ¾ cup of whole wheat flour
- ½ a tablespoon of baking powder
- 2 tablespoon of artificial sweetener
- ½ a tablespoon of cinnamon, ground
- 1 cup of skim milk
- 1 whole egg white, lightly beaten
- 1/3 cup of unsweetened applesauce

Directions

1. Take a bowl and add whole wheat flour, sugar substitute, baking powder, cinnamon
2. Take another bowl and add skim milk, egg white and apple sauce
3. Stir the flour mix into the egg mi and keep stirring until no lumps are present, the batter will be thick
4. Take a large skillet and place it over medium heat
5. Grease with cooking spray
6. Spoon two heaping tablespoon of batter (per cake) and spread it out lightly
7. Cook until both sides of the cake are golden brown
8. Serve and enjoy!

Nutrition Values (Per Serving)

- Calories: 210
- Fat: 1g
- Carbohydrates: 43g
- Protein: 11g

CHAPTER 3: LUNCH RECIPES

1. AMAZING BERRY BALSAMIC CHICKEN

(Prepping time: 10 minutes\ Cooking time: 35 minutes |For 4 servings\SmartPoints:3)

Ingredients

- 3 boneless chicken breast, skinless
- Salt and pepper as needed
- ¼ cup of all-purpose flour
- 2/3 cup of low fat chicken broth
- 1 and a ½ teaspoon of corn starch
- ½ a cup of low sugar raspberry preserve
- 1 and a ½ tablespoon of balsamic vinegar

Directions

1. Cut the chicken breast into bite sized portions and season with salt and pepper. Dredge the meat in flour and shake off any excess
2. Take a non-stick skillet and place it over medium heat
3. Add chicken and cook for 15 minutes, making sure to turn once halfway through. Remove chicken and transfer to a platter
4. Add cornstarch, broth, raspberry preserve into the same skillet and stir
5. Stir in balsamic vinegar and keep the heat on medium, stir cook for a few minutes
6. Transfer the chicken back to the skillet and cook for 15 minutes more, turning once. Serve and enjoy!

Nutrition Values (Per Serving)

- Calories: 546
- Fat: 35g
- Carbohydrates: 11g
- Protein: 44g

2. Slowly Cooked Hearty Chicken and Carrot Stew

(Prepping time: 20 minutes\ Cooking time: 6 hours |For 6 servings\SmartPoints:3)

Ingredients

- 4 boneless chicken breast, cubed
- 3 cups of carrots, peeled and cubed
- 1 cup onion, chopped
- 1 cup tomatoes, chopped
- 1 teaspoon of dried thyme
- 2 cups of chicken broth
- 2 garlic cloves, minced
- Salt and pepper as needed

Directions

1. Add all of the listed ingredients to a Slow Cooker
2. Stir and close the lid
3. Cook for 6 hours
4. Serve hot and enjoy!

Nutrition Values (Per Serving)

- Calories: 182
- Fat: 3g
- Carbohydrates: 10g
- Protein: 39g

3. Greek Lemon And Chicken Soup

(Prepping time: 15 minutes\ Cooking time: 30 minutes |For 4 servings\SmartPoints:2)

Ingredients

- 2 cups cooked chicken, chopped
- 2 medium carrots, chopped
- ½ a cup of onion, chopped
- ¼ cup lemon juice
- 1 clove garlic, minced
- 1 can cream of chicken soup, fat-free and low sodium
- 2 cans of chicken broth, fat free
- ¼ teaspoon of ground black pepper
- 2/3 cup of long-grain rice
- 2 tablespoon of parsley, snipped

Directions

1. Add all of the listed ingredients to a pot (except rice and parsley)
2. Season with salt and pepper
3. Bring the mix to a boil over medium-high heat
4. Stir in rice and set heat to medium
5. Simmer for 20 minutes until rice is tender
6. Garnish parsley and enjoy!

Nutrition Values (Per Serving)

- Calories: 582
- Fat: 33g
- Carbohydrates: 35g
- Protein: 32 g

4. Mouthwatering Broccoli And Cheese Soup

(Prepping time: 10 minutes\ Cooking time: 35 minutes |For 10 servings\SmartPoints:3)

Ingredients

- 3 can of 14 and ½ ounce (each) chicken broth
- 2 bag (1 pound each) frozen broccoli
- 1 can of 10 and a ½ ounce (each) tomatoes and green chili pepper
- 10 ounce Velveeta low fat cheese

Directions

1. Take a pot and add broth, frozen broccoli, tomatoes and chili
2. Mix well and place it over medium-high heat
3. Allow the mixture to heat up and reach a boil
4. Lower down the heat to low and simmer for 25 minutes until the veggies are tender
5. Cube Velveeta and drop them into the soup
6. Simmer until the cheese melts
7. Serve and enjoy!

Nutrition Values (Per Serving)

- Calories: 112
- Fat: 4g
- Carbohydrates: 9g
- Protein: 11g

5. Stir Fried Chicken

(Prepping time: 20 minutes\ Cooking time: 25 minutes |For 10 servings\SmartPoints:5)

Ingredients

- 2 and a ½ pounds of skinless, boneless chicken breast, sliced thin
- 4 tablespoon of fish sauce
- 2 teaspoon of Swerve
- 2 onions, thinly sliced
- 8 scallions, sliced
- ½ a cup of fresh cilantro, chopped
- 4 tablespoon of soy sauce
- 2 tablespoon of chili garlic sauce
- 4 tablespoon of olive oil
- 4 garlic cloves, minced
- Salt and pepper as needed

Directions

1. Take a bowl and add fish sauce, swerve, soy sauce and chili garlic sauce and mix well
2. Dredge the chicken in your sauce mix and let it marinate for 10 minutes
3. Take a large skillet and place it over medium- high heat
4. Add oil and allow the oil to heat up
5. Add onions and Saute for 4 minutes, add garlic and Saute for 1 minute more
6. Add chicken and marinade and Saute for 7 minutes
7. Add cilantro and scallions
8. Cook for 3 minutes more and stir in basil. Cook for 1 minute
9. Season with salt and pepper. Stir and enjoy!

Nutrition Values (Per Serving)

- Calories: 229
- Fat: 8g
- Carbohydrates: 10g
- Protein: 29g

6. Very Curious Mango Chicken

(Prepping time: 25 minutes\ Cooking time: 10 minutes |For 4 servings\SmartPoints:2)

Ingredients

- 2 medium mangoes, peeled and sliced
- 10 ounce coconut milk
- 4 teaspoon of vegetable oil
- 4 teaspoon of spicy curry paste
- 14 ounce chicken breast halves, skinless and boneless, cut in cubes
- 4 medium shallots
- 1 large English cucumber, sliced and seeded

Directions

1. Slice half of the mangoes and add the halves to a bowl
2. Add mangoes and coconut milk to a blender and blend until you have a smooth puree
3. Keep the mixture on the side
4. Tae a large sized pot and place it over medium heat, add oil and allow the oil to heat up
5. Add curry paste and cook for 1 minute until you have a nice fragrance, add shallots and chicken to the pot and cook for 5 minutes
6. Pour mango puree to the mix and allow it to heat up
7. Serve the cooked chicken with mango puree and cucumbers
8. Enjoy!

Nutrition Values (Per Serving)

- Calories: 398
- Fat: 20g
- Carbohydrates: 32g
- Protein: 26g

7. Squid and Egg Dish

(Prepping time: 15 minutes\ Cooking time: 10 minutes |For 6 servings\SmartPoints:5)

Ingredients

- 2 pounds squid, cleaned and cut into rings
- 2 eggs, beaten
- 2 teaspoon of olive oil
- ½ a yellow onion, sliced
- ½ a teaspoon of ground turmeric
- Salt as needed

Directions

1. Take a skillet and place it over medium-high heat
2. Add oil and allow the oil to heat up
3. Add onions and Saute for 5 minutes
4. Add turmeric and squid rings, season with salt
5. Simmer over medium-low heat for 5 minutes
6. Add beaten eggs
7. Cook for additional 3 minutes and serve immediately
8. Enjoy!

Nutrition Values (Per Serving)

- Calories: 178
- Fat: 6g
- Carbohydrates: 6g
- Protein: 25g

8. Olive and Tomato Salad

(Prepping time: 15 minutes\ Cooking time: 0 minutes |For 10 servings\SmartPoints:4)

Ingredients

- 1 can (2 and a ¼ ounce) green olives, pitted and chopped
- ¼ cup of red wine vinegar
- 5 large tomatoes, chopped
- ½ a red onion, sliced thinly
- 5 cucumbers, chopped
- 4 ounce feta cheese, crumbled
- 1 - 5 ounce can of black olives, pitted and halved

Directions

1. Add all of the listed ingredients to a large bowl (except vinegar) and mix well
2. Drizzle vinegar on top
3. Serve and enjoy!

Nutrition Values (Per Serving)

- Calories: 178
- Fat: 6g
- Carbohydrates: 6g
- Protein: 25g

9. Jalapeno Chicken "Grilled" Platter

(Prepping time: 5 minutes\ Cooking time: 10 minutes |For 4 servings\SmartPoints:5)

Ingredients

- 1/3 cup of steak sauce
- 1/3 cup of jalapeno jelly, melted
- 2 tablespoon of low-sodium Worcestershire sauce
- 1 teaspoon of garlic powder
- 4 pieces of 4 ounce (each) chicken breast halves, boneless and skinless

Directions

1. Take a large zip bag and add steak sauce, jelly ,Worcestershire sauce, garlic powder and add chicken
2. Seal the bag and shake until the chicken is coated well
3. Marinate in your fridge for at least 8 hours
4. Remove the chicken and discard the marinade
5. Coat a grill rack with cooking spray and pre-heat your grill to 350-400 degree Fahrenheit
6. Put chicken on grill rack and grill for 5 minutes each side
7. Serve and enjoy!

Nutrition Values (Per Serving)

- Calories: 202
- Fat: 1g
- Carbohydrates: 20g
- Protein: 26g

10. Caramelized Pork Chops And Onion

(Prepping time: 5 minutes\ Cooking time: 40 minutes |For 4 servings\SmartPoints:3)

Ingredients

- 4 pound chuck roast
- 4 ounce green Chili, chopped
- 2 tablespoon of chili powder
- ½ a teaspoon of dried oregano
- ½ a teaspoon of cumin, ground
- 2 garlic cloves, minced
- Salt as needed

Directions

1. Rub the chops with seasoning of 1 teaspoon of pepper and 2 teaspoon of salt
2. Take a skillet and place it over medium heat, add oil and allow the oil to heat up
3. Brown the seasoned chop both sides
4. Add water and onion to the skillet and cover, lower down the heat to low and simmer for 20 minutes
5. Turn the chops over and season with more salt and pepper
6. Cover and cook until the water fully evaporates and the beef shows a slightly brown texture
7. Remove the chops and serve with a topping of the caramelized onion. Serve and enjoy!

Nutrition Values (Per Serving)

- Calories: 47
- Fat: 4g
- Carbohydrates: 4g
- Protein: 0.5g

11. DIJON DRESSED FISH FILLETS

(Prepping time: 3 minutes\ Cooking time: 12 minutes |For 4 servings\SmartPoints:2)

Ingredients

- 1 and a ½ pound of fresh tilapia fillets
- ¼ cup of white cornmeal
- ¼ cup of dry seasoned bread crumbs
- ½ a teaspoon of dried dill
- ½ a teaspoon of salt
- 1/8 teaspoon of black pepper
- ½ a teaspoon of paprika
- 1/3 cup of skim milk
- 3 tablespoon of butter, melted

Directions

1. Pre-heat your oven to 450 degree Fahrenheit
2. Take an 11 x 7 inch baking dish and coat with cooking spray, arrange the fillets
3. Take a bowl and add mustard, lemon juice, Worcestershire sauce and stir
4. Spread the mix evenly over the fillets
5. Sprinkle breadcrumbs over the fillets as well
6. Bake for 12 minutes until the fish flakes when tested with fork
7. Cut fillet in half and serve
8. Enjoy!

Nutrition Values (Per Serving)

- Calories: 125
- Fat: 2g
- Carbohydrates: 6g
- Protein: 21g

12. Cool Orange Baked Chicken

(Prepping time: 10 minutes\ Cooking time: 35 minutes |For 4 servings\SmartPoints:2)

Ingredients

- 2 tablespoon of orange juice
- 2 tablespoon of Dijon mustard
- ¼ teaspoon of salt
- ¾ cup of crumbled whole wheat crackers
- 1 tablespoon of orange zest, grated
- 1 shallot, finely chopped
- ¼ teaspoon of black pepper, freshly ground
- 12 ounce chicken thigh, boneless and skinless

Directions

1. Pre-heat your oven to a temperature of 350 degree Fahrenheit
2. Take a non-stick baking sheet and spray it with cooking spray
3. Take a small bowl and combine orange juice, salt and mustard
4. Take a sheet of wax paper and combine cracker crumbs, shallot, orange zest and pepper
5. Brush up the chicken with the mustard mix and dredge the chicken in the crumbs
6. Firmly place the crumbs to coat all sides of the chicken
7. Place the chicken on your baking sheet
8. Bake for about 15 minutes, making sure to turn it over
9. Bake for another 15 minutes more. Serve!

Nutrition Values (Per Serving)

- Calories: 194
- Fat: 7g
- Carbohydrates: 15g
- Protein: 19g

13. Supreme Melon and Watercress Salad

(Prepping time: 10 minutes\ Cooking time: 0 minutes |For 4 servings\SmartPoints:1)

Ingredients

- 3 tablespoon of fresh lime juice
- 1 teaspoon of date paste
- 1 teaspoon of fresh ginger root, minced
- ¼ cup of olive oil
- 2 bunch of watercress, trimmed and chopped
- 2 and a ½ cups of watermelon, cubed
- 2 and a /12 cups of cantaloupe, cubed
- 1/3 cup almonds, toasted and sliced

Directions

1. Take a large sized bowl and add lime juice, date paste, ginger and whisk
2. Add olive oil and mix
3. Season with salt and pepper
4. Add watercress, cantaloupe and watermelon, toss well
5. Transfer to you serving bowl and garnish with sliced almonds
6. Enjoy!

Nutrition Values (Per Serving)

- Calories: 274
- Fat: 20g
- Carbohydrates: 21g
- Protein: 7g

14. Hearty Stir-Fried Shrimp

(Prepping time: 15 minutes\ Cooking time: 6 minutes |For 8 servings\SmartPoints:4)

Ingredients

- 1 pound raw jumbo shrimp, peeled and deveined
- 4 tablespoon of tamari
- 2 tablespoon of extra virgin olive oil
- 4 garlic cloves, minced
- Salt and pepper as needed

Directions

1. Take a large skillet and place it over medium heat
2. Add oil and allow the oil to heat up
3. Add garlic and Saute for 1 minute
4. Add tamari, salt, pepper and shrimp
5. Cook for about 5 minutes
6. Serve and enjoy!

Nutrition Values (Per Serving)

- Calories: 210
- Fat: 9g
- Carbohydrates: 4g
- Protein: 27g

15. Healthy Emmenthal Soup

(Prepping time: 5 minutes\ Cooking time: 5 minutes |For 2 servings\SmartPoints:1)

Ingredients

- 2 cups of cauliflower, small florets
- 1 whole potato, cubed
- 2 cups of yeast free vegetable stock
- 3 tablespoon of Emmenthal Cheese, cubed
- 2 tablespoon of fresh chives
- 2 tablespoon of pumpkin seeds
- 1 pinch of nutmeg
- 1 pinch of cayenne pepper

Directions

1. Take a pot and add vegetable broth, place it over medium heat and allow it to heat up
2. Add potatoes and cauliflower and cook them until tender
3. Transfer the veggies to a blender and puree
4. Return the pureed mixture to the broth and stir well
5. Season the soup with cayenne, nutmeg, salt and pepper
6. Add Emmenthal cheese, chives and stir
7. Garnish with pumpkin seed and enjoy!

Nutrition Values (Per Serving)

- Calories: 318
- Fat: 22g
- Carbohydrates: 16g
- Protein: 14g

CHAPTER 4: DINNER RECIPES

1. SIMPLE SOUR THAI SOUP

(Prepping time: 10 minutes\ Cooking time: 15 minutes |For 4 servings\SmartPoints:1)

Ingredients

- 3 cups of chicken stock
- 1 tablespoon of tom yum paste
- ½ a clove of garlic, finely chopped
- 3 stalks of lemon grass, chopped
- 2 kaffir lime leaves
- 2 skinless and boneless chicken breast, shredded
- 4 ounce mushrooms, thinly sliced
- 1 tablespoon of fish sauce
- 1 tablespoon of lime juice
- 1 teaspoon of chopped coriander
- 1 sprig fresh basil , chopped

Directions

1. Take a large sized saucepan and add chicken stock
2. Bring the stock to a boil
3. Add tom yum paste, garlic and cook for 2 minutes over medium heat
4. Stir in lemon grass, kaffir leaves and simmer over low heat for 5 minutes
5. Add mushrooms, fish sauce, lime juice, green chile, pepper and cook over medium heat until blended
6. Remove the heat and serve warm with a garnish of basil and coriander
7. Enjoy!

Nutrition Values (Per Serving)

- Calories: 71
- Fat: 1.8g
- Carbohydrates: 5g
- Protein: 10g

2. Potato And BBQ Chicken Slaw

(Prepping time: 5 minutes\ Cooking time: 45 minutes |For 2 servings\SmartPoints:2)

Ingredients

- 1 medium Sweet Potato
- 1 medium chicken breast, skinless and raw
- BBQ sauce as needed
- 1 tablespoon of low fat Mayonnaise
- 1 tablespoon of natural Greek Yogurt
- 1 teaspoon of fresh lemon juice
- 1 and a ¾ ounce of cabbage, shredded
- 1 ounce of raw carrots, grated
- 1 medium spring onion, sliced

Directions

1. Pre-heat your oven to 352 degree Fahrenheit
2. Prick the potato skin with fork and place them on a baking tray
3. Roast for 40-45 minutes
4. Take an oven proof dish and add chicken with 2 tablespoon of water
5. Cover with foil and bake for 25 minutes
6. Drain the cooking juice and cover chicken with BBQ sauce
7. Turn well to coat the chicken thoroughly
8. Cover again and bake for 15 minutes more
9. Take a bowl and add mayonnaise, yogurt, lemon juice and season with black pepper
10. Stir in cabbage, carrots and spring onion
11. Shred the chicken baked chicken using fork
12. Make a deep cut on top of the potato and fill it up with chicken
13. Serve with the Slaw and enjoy!

Nutrition Values (Per Serving)

- Calories: 472
- Fat: 26g
- Carbohydrates: 36g
- Protein: 24g

3. Asparagus And Scallops Medley

(Prepping time: 15 minutes\ Cooking time: 10 minutes |For 4 servings\SmartPoints:3)

Ingredients

- ¾ pound of baby scallops
- ¾ pound of fresh asparagus, trimmed and cut into 1 inch pieces
- 1 tablespoon of coconut oil
- 1 garlic clove, minced
- 1 teaspoon of fresh lemon zest, grated finely
- 1 tablespoon of fresh lemon juice
- 1/8 cup of shallots, chopped
- 1 tablespoon of fresh rosemary, chopped finely
- Salt and pepper as needed

Directions

1. Take a skillet and place it over medium-high heat
2. Add oil and allow the oil to heat up
3. Add shallots and Saute for 2 minutes
4. Add rosemary and garlic and Saute for 1 minute
5. Add lemon zest and asparagus
6. Cook for 2 minutes more and stir in scallops
7. Cook on medium-heat for 5 minutes
8. Drizzle lemon juice on top and season with salt and pepper
9. Serve and enjoy!

Nutrition Values (Per Serving)

- Calories: 150
- Fat: 5g
- Carbohydrates: 0.2g
- Protein: 26g

4. Goodnight Ginger And Salmon

(Prepping time: 20 minutes\ Cooking time: 18 minutes |For 6 servings\SmartPoints:4)

Ingredients

- ½ a pound of salmon fillets
- 1 tablespoon of coconut aminos
- ½ a tablespoon of fresh ginger, minced
- 1 tablespoon of sesame seeds
- Salt and pepper as needed

Directions

1. Pre-heat your oven to 325 degree Fahrenheit
2. Take a large baking sheet and grease it well
3. Take a bowl and add all of the ingredients except salmon
4. Dredge salmon in the mix and transfer salmon to your prepared baking sheet
5. Bake for 18 minutes
6. Serve hot and enjoy!

Nutrition Values (Per Serving)

- Calories: 192
- Fat: 10g
- Carbohydrates: 5g
- Protein: 22g

5. Prawn And Banana Salsa

(Prepping time: 15 minutes\ Cooking time: 3 minutes |For 4 servings\SmartPoints:2)

Ingredients

- 2 bananas, peeled and thinly sliced
- 2 cucumbers, peeled, seeded and diced
- ½ a cup of fresh mint leaves
- ½ a cup of fresh cilantro leaves
- 1 teaspoon of fresh ginger root, minced
- 1 red chile pepper, finely sliced
- ¼ cup of lime juice
- 1 tablespoon of fish sauce
- 1 tablespoon of brown sugar
- 1 and a ½ pound of tiger prawns, peeled and deveined

Directions

1. Take a large sized bowl and add bananas, cucumber, cilantro, ginger, red chile pepper and mix everything well
2. The above mix is your Salsa
3. Take a small sized bowl and add lime juice, brown sugar, fish sauce, sugar and blend. Add salsa mix to the fish sauce mix and stir
4. Take large saucepan and add salted water
5. Bring the water to a boil
6. Add prawns into the water and cook for 3 minutes
7. Serve the cooked prawn with banana salsa. Enjoy!

Nutrition Values (Per Serving)

- Calories: 280
- Fat: 2g
- Carbohydrates: 25g
- Protein: 36g

6. Daring Costa Brava Chicken

(Prepping time: 5 minutes\ Cooking time: 25 minutes |For 4 servings\SmartPoints:2)

Ingredients

- 1 can of 20 ounce Pineapple Chunks
- 10 chicken breast halves, skinless and boneless
- 1 tablespoon of vegetable oil
- 1 teaspoon of cumin, ground
- 1 teaspoon of cinnamon, ground
- 2 garlic cloves, minced
- 1 onion, quartered
- 1 can of 14 ounce stewed tomatoes
- 2 cups of black olives
- ½ a cup of salsa
- 2 tablespoon of water
- 1 red bell pepper, thinly sliced
- Salt as needed

Directions

1. Drain the pineapples and reserve the juice
2. Sprinkle with some salt
3. Take a large sized frying pan and place it over medium heat
4. Add oil and allow the oil to heat up
5. Add cinnamon, cumin and sprinkle it all over
6. Add garlic and onion and cook until tender
7. Add the reserved pineapple juice, salsa, olives and tomatoes
8. Cover it up and allow it to simmer for 25 minutes
9. Take a bowl and add cornstarch and water. Stir the mixture into pan
10. Add bell pepper and simmer for a little longer until the sauce boils and thickens
11. Stir in pineapple chunks and thoroughly heat it up. Enjoy

Nutrition Values (Per Serving)

- Calories: 239
- Fat: 6g
- Carbohydrates: 1g
- Protein: 28

7. Delightful Rosemary And Scallops

(Prepping time: 15 minutes\ Cooking time: 5 minutes |For 6 servings\SmartPoints:5)

Ingredients

- 2 pounds sea scallops
- 4 tablespoon of olive oil
- 4 tablespoon of fresh rosemary, chopped
- 4 garlic cloves, minced

Directions

1. Take skillet and place it over medium-high heat
2. Add oil allow the oil to heat up
3. Add garlic and rosemary
4. Saute for 1 minute
5. Add scallops and cook for 2 minutes (each side)
6. Serve and enjoy!

Nutrition Values (Per Serving)

- Calories: 223
- Fat: 10g
- Carbohydrates: 6g
- Protein: 25g

8. Bubbly Chicken Dish

(Prepping time: 15 minutes\ Cooking time: 30 minutes |For 4 servings\SmartPoints:5)

Ingredients

- 1 pack of 8 ounce biscuits
- 4 ounce soft light cream cheese
- 2 cups of cooked chicken, shredded
- 1/3 cup of light sour cream
- ¼ cup of ranch dressing
- 5 slices of bacon, cooked and crumbled
- ½ a cup of low fat cheese, shredded

Directions

1. Pre-heat your oven to 375 degree Fahrenheit
2. Take a 9x13 baking pan and grease it well
3. Cut biscuits and spread across bottom of the pan
4. Take a bowl and mix chicken, ranch dressing, sour cream, cream cheese
5. Spoon the mixture over biscuits and spread evenly
6. Bake for 30 minutes
7. Serve and enjoy!

Nutrition Values (Per Serving)

- Calories: 535
- Fat: 41g
- Carbohydrates: 22g
- Protein: 17g

9. Potato Crusted Herbed Tilapia

(Prepping time: 13 minutes\ Cooking time: 12 minutes |For 4 servings\SmartPoints:3)

Ingredients

- 3 tablespoon of light mayonnaise
- ½ a teaspoon of pickle relish
- ½ a teaspoon of lemon juice, freshly squeezed
- ½ a teaspoon of mustard, ground
- 2 tablespoon of green onions, chopped
- 4 pieces of 3 ounce tilapia fillets
- ½ a cup of potato flakes, organic
- Salt and pepper as needed
- ½ a cup of butter, melted

Directions

1. Pre-heat your oven to 450 degree Fahrenheit
2. Take a mixing bowl and add mayonnaise, pickle relish, mustard, lemon juice, onion and mix
3. Coat the fish fillets with the mixture and dredge the fillets on potato flakes
4. Press potato flakes into the tilapia and sprinkle salt and pepper
5. Place on your baking sheet and bake for 12 minutes
6. After the first 6 minutes, brush with butter
7. Serve and enjoy!

Nutrition Values (Per Serving)

- Calories: 354
- Fat: 30g
- Carbohydrates: 5g
- Protein: 18g

10. CRANBERRY CHICKEN DELUXE

(Prepping time: 20 minutes\ Cooking time: 20 minutes |For 3 servings\SmartPoints:4)

Ingredients

- ¾ pound of skinless, boneless chicken thigh
- 1 tablespoon of fresh ginger, minced
- ½ a cup of fresh cranberries
- 1 tablespoon of olive oil
- 1/8 cup of onion, chopped finely
- ½ a cup of chicken broth
- 1 tablespoon of unsweetened applesauce
- Salt and pepper as needed

Directions

1. Take a large skillet and place it over medium heat
2. Add oil and allow the oil to heat up
3. Add chicken, salt and black pepper
4. Cook for 5 minutes on each side
5. Transfer the cooked chicken to a large bowl
6. Put onions in the very skillet and Saute for 3 minutes
7. Stir in broth, cook for 5 minutes until boiled
8. Add cranberries and cook for 5 minutes
9. Drizzle applesauce and season with pepper and salt
10. Cook for 2 minutes more
11. Drizzle this cranberry mixture over your chicken. Serve and enjoy!

Nutrition Values (Per Serving)

- Calories: 185
- Fat: 7g
- Carbohydrates: 5g
- Protein: 25g

11. Bean And Turkey Wrap

(Prepping time: 20 minutes\ Cooking time: 13 minutes |For 6 servings\SmartPoints:3)

Ingredients

- 6 ounce lean ground turkey
- 3 tablespoon tomato sauce
- ¼ teaspoon of ground cumin
- ½ a cup of black beans, cooked
- 6 large butternut lettuce leaves
- 1/3 cup of onion, minced
- ¼ teaspoon of garlic powder
- 3 teaspoons of extra-virgin olive oil
- Salt and pepper as needed

Directions

1. Take a bowl and add turkey, sauce, cumin, onion, garlic powder, pepper and salt
2. Mix well
3. Take a large skillet and place it over medium-heat
4. Add oil and allow the oil to heat up
5. Add turkey mix cook thoroughly for 10 minutes
6. Stir in tomato and beans
7. Simmer for 3 minutes more and keep it on the side
8. Divide the turkey mix over lettuce wraps and serve
9. Enjoy!

Nutrition Values (Per Serving)

- Calories: 121
- Fat: 4g
- Carbohydrates: 11g
- Protein: 10g

12. Mouthwatering Piri-Piri Chicken

(Prepping time: 10 minutes\ Cooking time: 35 minutes |For 2 servings\SmartPoints:2)

Ingredients

- 6 ounce raw potato, cut in wedges
- Cooking spray as needed
- 1 medium chicken breast, skinless and raw
- 1 small sachet of Piri Piri sauce
- 1 medium corn on a cob
- 1 medium whole meal pitta bread
- 1 portion of vegetable salad of your choice
- 5 tablespoon of natural Greek yogurt
- 1 teaspoon of mint sauce

Directions

1. Preheat your oven to 392 degree Fahrenheit
2. Put wedges on a baking tray and mist with cooking spray
3. Bake for 35 minutes
4. Add chicken on a chopping board and slice the fillet half lengthwise, making sure to opening by the middle
5. Place Clingfilm on either side of the chicken and bash with a rolling pin
6. Transfer to a dish and cover with Piri Piri sauce
7. Keep it on the side and allow it to sit for 15 minutes
8. Take a nonstick frying pan and place it over medium heat
9. Mist with cooking spray
10. Add corn and cook for 10 minutes
11. Turn off until the kernels are slightly charred
12. Mist the pan with more cooking spray and add the chicken, cook for minutes making sure to turn it halfway until fully cooked

13. Sprinkle pitta with a few drops water and bake for 3-4 minutes until they puff up
14. Take another bowl and mix yogurt and mint sauce
15. Slice the chicken, split the pitta and fill the pita with chicken and salad
16. Drizzle yogurt dressing on top and serve with corn, salad and wedges
17. Enjoy!

Nutrition Values (Per Serving)

- Calories: 533
- Fat: 21g
- Carbohydrates: 54g
- Protein: 35g

13. Easy Grilled Cod

(Prepping time: 20 minutes\ Cooking time: 6 minutes |For 8 servings\SmartPoints:2)

Ingredients

- 8 cod fillets (4 ounce each)
- 1 teaspoon of red pepper flakes
- 2 tablespoon of olive oil
- 1 teaspoon of dried dill
- 2 tablespoon of fresh lime juice
- Salt and pepper as needed

Directions

1. Take a bowl and mix everything except cod
2. Dredge the cod in the mixture and keep the cod n the side
3. Allow them to marinate for about 30 minutes
4. Pre-heat your grill to medium-high and grease the grate
5. Grill the cod fillets for 4 minutes on each side and serve
6. Enjoy!

Nutrition Values (Per Serving)

- Calories: 150
- Fat: 5g
- Carbohydrates: 0.2g
- Protein: 26g

14. Southwestern Divine Pork Chops

(Prepping time: 2 minutes\ Cooking time: 13 minutes |For 4 servings\SmartPoints:3)

Ingredients

- Cooking spray as needed
- 4 ounce pork loin chop, boneless and fat rimmed
- 1/3 cup of salsa
- 2 tablespoon of fresh lime juice
- ¼ cup of fresh cilantro, chopped

Directions

1. Take a large sized non-stick skillet and spray it with cooking spray
2. Heat it up until hot over high eat
3. Press the chops with your palm to flatten them slightly
4. Add them to the skillet and cook on 1 minute for each side until they are nicely browned
5. Lower down the heat to medium-low
6. Combine the salsa and lime juice
7. Pour the mix over the chops
8. Simmer uncovered for about 8 minutes until the chops are perfectly done
9. If needed, sprinkle some cilantro on top
10. Serve!

Nutrition Values (Per Serving)

- Calories: 184
- Fat: 8g
- Carbohydrates: 2g
- Protein: 25g

15. Maple And Mustard Salmon

(Prepping time: 15 minutes\ Cooking time: 15 minutes |For 4 servings\SmartPoints:1)

Ingredients

- 1 and a ½ pounds of raw wild salmon
- 3 tablespoon of whole grain mustard
- 2 tablespoon of maple syrup
- Salt and pepper as needed

Directions

1. Pre-heat your oven to 350 degree Fahrenheit
2. Take a mixing bowl and add all of the listed ingredients (except salmon)
3. Add salmon to the mixture and coat it well
4. Transfer to baking sheet lined with foil
5. Bake for 15 minutes
6. Serve and enjoy!

Nutrition Values (Per Serving)

- Calories: 298
- Fat: 10g
- Carbohydrates: 11g
- Protein: 35g

16. Oven Fried Macho Fish

(Prepping time: 10 minutes\ Cooking time: 10 minutes |For 4 servings\SmartPoints:5)

Ingredients

- 1 and a ½ pound of fresh tilapia fillets
- ¼ cup of white cornmeal
- ¼ cup of dry seasoned bread crumbs
- ½ a teaspoon of dried dill
- ½ a teaspoon of salt
- 1/8 teaspoon of black pepper
- ½ a teaspoon of paprika
- 1/3 cup of skim milk
- 3 tablespoon of butter, melted

Directions

1. Pre-heat your oven to 450 degree Fahrenheit
2. Take a shallow dish and add all of the listed dry ingredients
3. Take another shallow dish and add milk
4. Dip fish in milk and then in the crumb mix
5. Take a coated (greased) baking pan and transfer the fish to the pan
6. Drizzle butter on top
7. Bake in your oven for 10 minutes until the fish flakes with a fork
8. Serve and enjoy!

Nutrition Values (Per Serving)

- Calories: 196
- Fat: 7g
- Carbohydrates: 8g
- Protein: 24g

17. Fine Smothered Pork Chops

(Prepping time: 15 minutes\ Cooking time: 30 minutes |For 4 servings\SmartPoints:6)

Ingredients

- 4 pork chops, bone-in
- 2 tablespoon of olive oil
- ¼ cup of vegetable broth
- ½ a pound of Yukon gold potatoes, peeled and chopped
- 1 large onion, sliced
- 2 garlic cloves, minced
- 2 teaspoon of rubbed sage
- 1 teaspoon of thyme, ground
- Salt and pepper as needed

Directions

1. Pre-heat your oven to 350 degree Fahrenheit
2. Take a large sized skillet and place it over medium heat
3. Add a tablespoon of oil and allow the oil to heat up
4. Add pork chops and cook them for 4-5 minutes per side until browned
5. Transfer chops to a baking dish
6. Pour broth over the chops
7. Add remaining oil to the pan and Saute potatoes, onion, garlic for 3-4 minutes
8. Take a large bowl and add potatoes, garlic, onion, thyme, sage, pepper and salt
9. Transfer this mixture to the baking dish (wish pork)
10. Bake for 20-30 minutes
11. Serve and enjoy!

Nutrition Values (Per Serving)

- Calories: 261
- Fat: 10g
- Carbohydrates: 1.3g
- Protein: 2gg

18. BLACK ZUCCHINI WRAPPED FISH

(Prepping time: 15 minutes\ Cooking time: 15 minutes |For 4 servings\SmartPoints:0)

Ingredients

- 24 ounce cod fillets, skin removed
- 1 tablespoon of blackening spices
- 2 zucchinis, sliced lengthwise from to form ribbon
- ½ a tablespoon of olive oil

Directions

1. Season the fish fillets with blackening spice
2. Wrap each fish fillets with zucchini ribbons
3. Place fish on a plate
4. Take a skillet and place it over medium heat
5. Pour oil and allow the oil to heat up
6. Add wrapped fish to the skillet and cook each side for 4 minutes
7. Serve and enjoy!

Nutrition Values (Per Serving)

- Calories: 397
- Fat: 23g
- Carbohydrates: 2g
- Protein: 46g

19. Fine And Dandy BBQ Meatloaf

(Prepping time: 5 minutes\ Cooking time: 40 minutes |For 4 servings\SmartPoints:6)

Ingredients

- 1 pound 93% lean ground beef
- ½ a cup of BBQ sauce
- ¼ cup of frozen chopped onion, pressed dry
- ¼ cup of seasoned Italian bread crumbs
- 2 large egg whites

Directions

1. Pre-heat your oven to 375 degree Fahrenheit
2. Take a bowl and add meat, ¼ cup of BBQ sauce, onion, egg whites, bread crumbs, seasoning of your choice
3. Stir
4. Shape the mixture into a loaf pan
5. Spread remaining ¼ cup of BBQ sauce over loaf
6. Bake for 40 minutes at 375 degree Fahrenheit
7. Check the doneness and enjoy!

Nutrition Values (Per Serving)

- Calories: 240
- Fat: 6g
- Carbohydrates: 17g
- Protein: 27g

20. Turtle Munchies Salad

(Prepping time: 5 minutes\ Cooking time: 0 minutes |For 2 servings\SmartPoints:1)

Ingredients

- 1 Romaine lettuce, chopped
- 3 Roma tomatoes, diced
- 1 English cucumber, diced
- 1 small red onion, diced
- ½ a cup of curly parsley, chopped
- 2 tablespoon of virgin olive oil
- ½ a large lemon, juiced
- 1 teaspoon of garlic powder
- Salt and pepper as needed

Directions

1. Wash the vegetables well under cold water
2. Chop, diced and mince them accordingly
3. Take a large salad bowl and transfer the vegetables
4. Add vegetable oil, olive oil , lemon juice and other spices
5. Toss well and chill
6. Serve and enjoy!

Nutrition Values (Per Serving)

- Calories: 200
- Fat: 8g
- Carbohydrates: 18g
- Protein: 10g

21. Turkey and Peas Medley

(Prepping time: 20 minutes\ Cooking time: 60 minutes |For 3 servings\SmartPoints:5)

Ingredients

- ½ a medium onion, chopped
- 3 garlic cloves, minced
- ¼ teaspoon of ground cumin
- ¼ teaspoon of ground nutmeg
- ½ a pound of lean ground turkey
- 1 cup water
- ¼ cup of fresh cilantro, chopped
- ¾ cup of fresh green peas, shelled
- 1 bay leaf
- ¼ cup of fresh tomatoes, chopped
- 1 bay leaf
- ¼ teaspoon of ground turmeric
- 1 teaspoon of ground coriander
- ¼ teaspoon of fresh ginger, minced
- ½ a tablespoon of olive oil
- Salt and pepper as needed

Directions

1. Take a large pan and place it over medium heat
2. Add oil and allow the oil to heat up
3. Add onions and Saute for 4 minutes
4. Add spices, garlic cloves, ginger and Saute for 2 minutes more
5. Add turkey and cook for 6 minutes
6. Add tomatoes and cook for 9 minutes
7. Add water and green peas and cook for 30 minutes more
8. Remove the heat and season with salt and pepper
9. Garnish with cilantro and enjoy!

Nutrition Values (Per Serving)

- Calories: 175
- Fat: 9g
- Carbohydrates: 10g
- Protein: 17

22. Hearty Cabbage Soup

(Prepping time: 7 minutes\ Cooking time: 25 minutes |For 6 servings\SmartPoints:1)

Ingredients

- 3 cups non-fat beef stock
- 2 garlic cloves, minced
- 1 tablespoon of tomato paste
- 2 cup cabbage, chopped
- ½ a yellow onion
- ½ a cup carrot, chopped
- ½ a cup green beans
- ½ a cup zucchini, chopped
- ½ a teaspoon of basil
- ½ a teaspoon of oregano
- Salt and pepper as needed

Directions

1. Grease a pot with non-stick cooking spray
2. Place it over medium heat and allow the oil the heat up
3. Add onions, carrots and garlic and Saute for 5 minutes
4. Add broth, tomato paste, green beans, cabbage, basil, oregano, salt and pepper
5. Bring the whole mix to a boil and lower down the heat, simmer for 5-10 minutes until all veggies are tender
6. Add zucchini and simmer for 5 minutes more. Sever hot and enjoy!

Nutrition Values (Per Serving)

- Calories: 22
- Fat: 0g
- Carbohydrates: 5g
- Protein: 1g

23. Raspberry And Chicken Supreme

(Prepping time: 10 minutes\ Cooking time: 20 minutes |For 4 servings\SmartPoints:4)

Ingredients

- 3 pieces of chicken breast, skinless and boneless
- Salt and pepper as needed
- ¼ cup of all-purpose flour
- 2/3 cup of low-fat chicken broth
- 1 and a ½ teaspoon of corn starch
- ½ a cup of low sugar raspberry preserve
- 1 and a ½ tablespoon of balsamic vinegar

Directions

1. Cut the chicken into bite sized portions and season with salt and pepper
2. Dredge the chicken in flour and shake off any excess
3. Take a non-stick skillet and place it over medium heat
4. Add chicken and cook for 15 minutes, making sure to turn them over halfway through Add corn starch, chicken broth, raspberry preserve to a skillet and place it over medium heat, stir in vinegar
5. Add chicken pieces to the skillet and cook for 15 minutes more making sure to turn them halfway through
6. Serve and enjoy!

Nutrition Values (Per Serving)

- Calories: 546
- Fat: 35g
- Carbohydrates:11g
- Protein: 44g

CHAPTER 5: DESSERT RECIPES

1. AUTHENTIC BANANA CUSTARD

(Prepping time: 20 minutes\ Cooking time: 25 minutes |For 8 servings\SmartPoints:2)

Ingredients

- 2 ripe bananas, peeled and mashed finely
- ½ a teaspoon of vanilla extract
- 14 ounce unsweetened almond milk
- 3 eggs

Directions

1. Pre-heat your oven to 350 degree Fahrenheit
2. Grease 8 custard glasses lightly
3. Arrange the glasses in a large baking dish
4. Take a large bowl and mix all of the ingredients and mix them well until combined nicely
5. Divide the mixture evenly between the glasses
6. Pour water in the baking dish
7. Bake for 25 minutes
8. Take it out and serve
9. Enjoy!

Nutrition Values (Per Serving)

- Calories: 59
- Fat: 2.4g
- Carbohydrates: 7g
- Protein: 3g

2. Curious Blackberry Crumble

(Prepping time: 20 minutes\ Cooking time: 45 minutes |For 8 servings\SmartPoints:4)

Ingredients

- ½ a cup of coconut flour
- ½ a cup of banana, peeled and mashed
- 6 tablespoon of water
- 3 cups of fresh blackberries
- ½ a cup of arrowroot flour
- 1 and a ½ teaspoon of baking soda
- 4 tablespoon of butter, melted
- 1 tablespoon of fresh lemon juice

Directions

1. Pre-heat your oven to 300 degree Fahrenheit
2. Take a baking dish and grease it lightly
3. Take a bowl and mix all of the ingredients except black berries, mix well
4. Place blackberries in the bottom of your baking dish and top with flour
5. Bake for 40 minutes
6. Serve and enjoy!

Nutrition Values (Per Serving)

- Calories: 92
- Fat: 7g
- Carbohydrates: 9g
- Protein: 8g

3. Unique Carrot Balls

(Prepping time: 10 minutes\ Cooking time: 0 minutes |For 10 servings\SmartPoints:2)

Ingredients

- 6 Mejdool dates, pitted
- 1 carrot, finely grated
- ¼ cup of raw walnuts
- ¼ cup of unsweetened coconut, shredded
- 1 teaspoon of nutmeg
- 1/8 teaspoon of salt

Directions

1. Take a food processor and add dates, ¼ cup of grated carrots, salt coconut , nutmeg
2. Mix well and puree the mixture
3. Add the walnuts and remaining ¼ cup of carrots
4. Pulse the mixture until you have a clunky texture
5. Form balls using your hand and roll them up in coconut
6. Top with carrots and chill
7. Enjoy!

Nutrition Values (Per Serving)

- Calories: 326
- Fat: 16g
- Carbohydrates: 42g
- Protein: 3g

4. The Lover's Blueberry Pudding

(Prepping time: 20 minutes\ Cooking time: 0 minutes |For 6 servings\SmartPoints:6)

Ingredients

- 2 cups of frozen blueberries
- 2 teaspoon of lime zest, grated freshly
- 20 drops of liquid stevia
- 2 small avocados, peeled, pitted and chopped
- ½ a teaspoon of fresh ginger, grated freshly
- 4 tablespoon of fresh lime juice
- 10 tablespoon of water

Directions

1. Add all of the listed ingredients to a blender (except blueberries) and pulse the mixture well
2. Transfer the mix into small serving bowls and chill the bowls
3. Serve with a topping of blueberries
4. Enjoy!

Nutrition Values (Per Serving)

- Calories: 166
- Fat: 13g
- Carbohydrates: 13g
- Protein: 1.7g

5. HUMMING YOGURT CHEESECAKE

(Prepping time: 20 minutes\ Cooking time: 35 minutes |For 5 servings\SmartPoints:3)

Ingredients

- 3 drops of liquid stevia
- ¼ cup of raw cacao powder
- ½ a teaspoon of vanilla extract
- 1 and a ½ cups of low fat Greek Yogurt
- 2 egg whites
- 1/8 cup of arrowroot starch
- Pinch of salt

Directions

1. Pre-heat your oven to 350 degree Fahrenheit
2. Grease a 9 inch cake pan
3. Take a large bowl and add all of the ingredients, mix well to form the batter
4. Transfer the batter into the pan and spread it out evenly
5. Bake for 35 minutes
6. Refrigerate for 4 hours and cut into equal sized slices
7. Serve and enjoy!

Nutrition Values (Per Serving)

- Calories: 85
- Fat: 1.6g
- Carbohydrates: 10g
- Protein: 7g

6. EXTREME WATERMELON SORBET

(Prepping time: 10 minutes\ Chill time: 20 hours |For 4 servings\SmartPoints:2)

Ingredients

- 4 cups watermelons, seedless and chunked
- ¼ cup of superfine sugar
- 2 tablespoon of lime juice

Directions

1. Add the listed ingredients to a blender and puree
2. Transfer to a freezer container with tight fitting lid
3. Freeze the mix for about 4-6 hours until you have a gelatin like consistency
4. Puree the mix once again in batches and return to the container
5. Chill overnight
6. Allow the sorbet to stand for 5 minutes before serving and enjoy!

Nutrition Values (Per Serving)

- Calories:91
- Fat: 0g
- Carbohydrates: 25g
- Protein: 1g

7. Heart Throb Chocolate and Tofu Mousse

(Prepping time: 180 minutes\ Cooking time: 0 minutes |For 4 servings\SmartPoints:3)

Ingredients

- 1 and a ½ medium bananas, peeled and sliced
- 2 teaspoon of cocoa powder
- 12 ounce firm tofu, drained
- 2 teaspoon of almonds

Directions

1. Add all of the listed ingredients to a food processor and pulse until you have a smooth mixture
2. Transfer the mixture to serving glasses and chill for 3 hours
3. Serve and enjoy!

Nutrition Values (Per Serving)

- Calories: 107
- Fat: 4g
- Carbohydrates: 12g
- Protein: 8g

8. Just 4 Ingredients Guacamole

(Prepping time: 10 minutes\ Cooking time: 0 minutes |For 12 servings\SmartPoints:2)

Ingredients

- 2 avocado, peeled, pitted and chopped
- 1 plum tomato, chopped
- 2 tablespoon of onion, finely chopped
- ¼ teaspoon of salt

Directions

1. Take a medium sized bowl and add avocado
2. Gently mash it until chunky
3. Stir in tomato, onion and salt
4. Serve as a dipper for your favorite crisp or vegetable bites!
5. Enjoy!

Nutrition Values (Per Serving)

- Calories: 55
- Fat: 5g
- Carbohydrates: 3g
- Protein: 1g

9. MAGNIFICENT APPLE AND OATMEAL MUFFINS

(Prepping time: 10 minutes\ Cooking time: 15 minutes |For 12 servings\SmartPoints:6)

Ingredients

- 2 cups of apple, peeled and shredded
- 1 and a ½ cups of all-purpose flour
- 1 cup of quick cooking oats
- 2/3 cup of brown sugar, firmly packed
- 1 and a ½ teaspoon of baking powder
- ½ a teaspoon of baking soda
- ½ a teaspoon of salt
- ½ a teaspoon of cinnamon, ground
- ½ a cup of milk
- 2 tablespoon of vegetable oil

Directions

1. Pre-heat your oven to 375 degree Fahrenheit
2. Take 12 muffin cups and line them with paper liners
3. Take a bowl and add flour, oats, brown sugar, baking so da, baking powder, salt, milk, cinnamon and oil
4. Mix well until the batter forms
5. Divide the batter between the muffin cups
6. Bake for 15-18 minutes until a toothpick comes out clean
7. Serve and enjoy!

Nutrition Values (Per Serving)

- Calories: 167
- Fat: 3g
- Carbohydrates: 32g
- Protein: 3g

10. Broccoli Cheddar And Egg Muffin

(Prepping time: 10 minutes\ Cooking time: 15 minutes |For 12 servings\SmartPoints:4)

Ingredients

- 2 green onions, chopped
- ¾ cup low fat shredded cheddar cheese
- 2 cups of broccoli, steamed and chopped
- Salt and pepper as needed
- ½ a tablespoon of Dijon mustard
- 4 egg whites
- 8 whole eggs

Directions

1. Lightly grease you muffin tins with cooking spray
2. Pre-heat your oven to 350 degree Fahrenheit
3. Take a bowl and whisk in eggs, egg whites, salt, pepper and mustard
4. Add remaining ingredients to the batter and whisk
5. Pour batter and divide between the muffin tins
6. Bake in your oven for 12 minutes until the center is puffy
7. Serve and enjoy!

Nutrition Values (Per Serving)

- Calories: 73
- Fat: 5g
- Carbohydrates: 2g
- Protein: 6g

11. No Cook PB And Oats

(Prepping time: 5 minutes\ Cooking time: 0 minutes |For 6 servings\SmartPoints:7)

Ingredients

- 1 tablespoon of sugar free jam
- 1 tablespoon of peanut butter
- ¾ cup of almond milk
- ½ a cup of old-fashioned oats

Directions

7. Take a bowl and add all of the listed ingredients (except jam)
8. Cover and keep it in the fridge
9. Enjoy the mix with a tablespoon of jam
10. Enjoy!

Nutrition Values (Per Serving)

- Calories: 243
- Fat: 11g
- Carbohydrates: 35g
- Protein: 6g

THE FINAL WORDS

I would like to take a moment of your time and thank you for reading the book to the end! I really do hope that you enjoyed the contents of this book and found the information to be useful and helpful.

Just like all diets out there, The effectiveness of the Weight Watchers Freestyle will also depend on how much sincerely you are following the given set of rules and how devoted you are to the cause.

It's not possible to change the dietary mistakes that we made in the past, but with the help of my book and the SmartPoints system of the Weight Watcher Freestyle, I hope that you attain a brighter and healthier future!

Stay safe and God Bless!

15791457R00049

Printed in Great Britain
by Amazon